Ketogenic Diet

Comprehensive Beginner's Guide to Ketogenic Diet

The Health Buff

The information provided in this book is designed to provide helpful information on the subjects discussed. The author's books are only meant to provide the reader with the basics knowledge of the topic in question, without any warranties regarding whether the reader will, or will not, be able to incorporate and apply all the information provided. Although the writer will make his best effort share her insights, the topic in question is a complex one, and each person needs a different timeframe to fully incorporate new information. Neither this book, nor any of the author's books constitute a promise that the reader will learn anything within a certain timeframe.

Table Of Contents

Introduction to Ketogenic Diet

A Ketogenic Diet is a very high-fat and low-carb diet. Keto is short for the state of ketosis that happens when most of the body's energy comes from ketone bodies in the blood than from glucose obtained from eating foods with more carbohydrates. Ketosis only takes place when fat provides your body's daily calorie needs, which takes the place of glucose as the best source of bodily energy.

While you're on a ketogenic diet, you need to avoid eating all or most foods with sugar and starch as they all have high carb content. These foods are broken down into sugar in our blood once we eat them, and if these levels become too high, more calories are easily stored as body fat and will resultan unwanted weight gain. However, when glucose levels dropped due to ketogenic dieting, the body will start to burn fat instead and produces ketones that can be measured in the blood.

Types of Ketogenic Diets

Ketogenic diets are generally believed as low carb and high fat diets similar to Atkins diet, but there are other variations which can make the diet better for you depending on your body's condition.

This book willhelp you differentiatethe types ofketogenic diets and help you decide which one is right for you.

- Standard Ketogenic Diet (SKD)

SKD is the type that most people follow as it is what's effective on them. It focuses on the high consumption of healthy fats or the 70% of your diet, 25% moderate protein, and 5% of carbohydrates.

- Targeted Ketogenic Diet (TKD)

TKD is almost the same as the SKD. They only vary on the permitted carbohydrates that require a workout. In this method, you are allowed to eat the entirety of your allotted carbs for the day in one meal at least 60 minutes before you exercise. The idea here is to use the energy from the carbs that you take effectively before it disrupts ketosis.

If you're following this approach, it might help if you eat carbs that are easily digestible with a high glycemic index to avoid upsetting your stomach. Then, when you're done exercising, increase your intake of protein to help with your muscle recovery, and thenyou can continue consuming your fats afterwards.

- Cyclic Ketogenic Diet (CKD)

CKD is a Cycle between a normal ketogenicdiet, followed by a set number of days of high carb intake. The idea is that it helps retain lean mass and it also makes the diet easier to live with.

Benefits of the Ketogenic Diet

- Weight Loss

If you're trying to lose weight, then a ketogenic diet might be one of the best ways to do it as it helps access and shed your body fats effectively. Obese people in particular can significantly benefit from this method.

- Reducing Appetite

Constant hunger can cause you to eat more food that has more calorie content that are difficult to burn and can eventually lead to weight gain. A ketogenic diet can help you avoid this problem as reducing your carb consumption can reduce hunger.

- Lowering Insulin Levels

When you consume lots of carbohydrates, they are broken down into sugars in the digestive tract and cause your blood sugar levels to rise and leads to a spike in your insulin. Overtime, you may develop major problem on your system like the insulin resistance.

This problem can lead totype2 diabetes when your body fails to secrete enough insulin to lower the blood sugar after meals.

By changing your diet to a ketogenic approach, you can reduce your risk of developing type 2 diabetes.

In one study in type 2 diabetes, 95.2% had managed to reduce or eliminate their glucose-lowering medication within 6 months by lowering their carb consumption.

- Lowering the Risk of Cancer

One of the good discoveries about the ketogenic diet is how it can help to prevent or lower the risk of cancer. Dominic D'Agostino, Ph.D., an assistant professor at the University of South Florida has test and developednutritional and metabolic therapies which include the ketogenic diet that can help control this disease.

D'Agostino explains that allour cells use glucose as fuel. However, the cancer cells do not have metabolic flexibility to adapt in using ketones as energy, which our regular cells can. Once the body enters a state of nutritional ketosis, the cancer cells will die.

What to Eat:

- Seafood
- Low-Carb Vegetables
- Cheese
- Avocados
- Eggs
- Meat and Poultry
- Coconut Oil
- Plain Greek Yogurt and Cottage Cheese
- Olive Oil
- Nuts and Seeds
- Berries
- Butter and Cream

What to Avoid:

- Artificial Sweeteners
- Milk
- Alcoholic and Sweet Drinks
- Tropical Fruit
- Soy Products
- All Grains
- Factory-farmed Pork and Fish
- Processed Foods
- Wheat
- Oats
- Rice
- Corn
- Green peas
- Sweet potatoes
- Potatoes
- Peas
- Cane sugar
- Breads made from any of the above
- Pastas made from any of the above

To help you get started with your Keto Diet, we listedseveral recipes to make sure that you're doing it the right way. But always remember to ask for a supervision of a doctor or a dietitian to avoid any health issues in the future.

THE

RECIPES

BREAKFAST RECIPES

TASTY CINNAMON TOASTS

Serving: 1

PrepTime: 5 Min

Ingredients:

- ½ teaspoon ground cinnamon
- ⅛ teaspoon ground nutmeg
- ¼ teaspoon sea salt
- 1 cup crushed pork rinds
- ¼ cup organic heavy whipping cream
- 2 drops liquid vanilla stevia

Instruction:

1. Get a small bowl and stir together the heavy cream, vanilla stevia, cinnamon, nutmeg, and salt. Then add and stir in the pork rinds.
2. Serve and enjoy!

CINNAMON EGGS

Serving: 2

PrepTime: 15 Min

Ingredients:

- 1 tablespoon Sugar-Free Vanilla Bean Sweetener
- ⅛ teaspoon ground cinnamon
- 4 large free-range eggs, hardboiled and peeled
- 2 tablespoons mayonnaise

Instruction:

1. Separate the yolks into a small bowl then place the egg white on a plate.
2. Add the mayonnaise, sweetener and cinnamon to the yolks and mix them together.
3. Transfer the egg yolk mixture to a zip lock plastic bag and cut off a small portion of the bag on the bottom. Pipe some of the mixture into each egg white.
4. Serve and enjoy!

CINNAMON WITH VANILLA &COCONUT CEREALS

Serving: 4

PrepTime: 5 Min

CookTime: 5 Min

Ingredients:

- Ground cinnamon
- Powdered stevia
- Unsweetened almond milk
- 2 cups unsweetened shaved coconut
- ½ cup crushed walnuts
- 1 vanilla bean, seeds scraped out

Instruction:

1. Preheat the oven to 350°F.
2. Prepare a rimmed baking sheet with parchment paper.
3. Put the coconut and walnuts in an even layer on the prepared sheet, spread them evenly then toast for about 5 minutes.

4. Once done, sprinkle them with vanilla bean seeds, cinnamon, and stevia.

5. Put ½ cup of cereal in a bowl and pour in your ideal amount of unsweetened almond milk. Serve immediately.

RICOTTA PANCAKES WITH LEMON &LAVENDER

Serving: 2
PrepTime: 5 Min
CookTime: 10 Min

Ingredients:

- 1 tablespoon organic culinary lavender
- ½ teaspoon baking powder
- 1 tablespoon Ghee
- Grated zest of 1 Meyer lemon
- Grass-fed butter
- Sugar-free maple syrup
- 4 large free-range eggs
- ¼ cup organic ricotta cheese
- 2 teaspoons Sugar-Free Vanilla Bean Sweetener
- 1 teaspoon freshly squeezed Meyer lemon juice
- 2 tablespoons coconut flour

Instruction:

1. Combine the eggs, ricotta cheese, sweetener, lemon juice, coconut flour, lavender, and baking powder in a blender then blend for 10 seconds.
2. In a medium pan, melt the ghee over medium heat. Pour at least ¼ cup of the butter into the pan.
3. Cook the pancake for 1 minute or until the bottom is crispy. Flip the pancake and cook for 1 minute more. Repeat this step to cook more pancakes.
4. Sprinkle each serving with lemon zest and top the pancakes with butter.
5. Serve with your favorite sugar-free maple syrup.

RICOTTA OATMEAL

Serving: 1

PrepTime: 5 Min

CookTime: 1 Min

Ingredients:

- ⅛ teaspoon ground cinnamon
- Sweetener to taste
- ½ cup organic ricotta cheese
- 4 tablespoons salted grass-fed butter

Instruction:

1. In a small microwave-safe bowl, mix the ricotta cheese, cinnamon, butter and sweetener. Heat it for about 1 minute.

CAJUN CAULIFLOWER HASH EGGS

Serving: 4

PrepTime: 10 Min

CookTime: 20 Min

Ingredients:

- 8 ounces shaved pastrami, chopped
- ½ green bell pepper, chopped
- 2 tablespoons minced garlic
- 1 teaspoon Cajun seasoning
- 1 bag frozen cauliflower florets
- 2 tablespoons extra-virgin olive oil
- ½ sweet yellow onion, chopped
- 4 large free-range eggs, lightly beaten

Instruction:

1. Steam the caulifowerfor about 6 minutes.
2. Drain the cauliflower and chop it into small pieces.

3. In a medium pan, heat the olive oil over medium heat.
4. Add the onion and sauté for about 3 to 5 minutes.
5. Add the eggs to the pan and gently stir for 2 minutes.
6. Add in and stir the cauliflower, green bell pepper, garlic, pastrami and Cajun seasoning into the scrambled eggs and onion.
7. Continue cooking the mixture for 5 minutes more.
8. Serve immediately and enjoy!

SPICY PULLED PORK EGGS BENEDICT

Serving: 1
PrepTime: 10 Min
CookTime: 3 Min

Ingredients:

- ➢ **ForTheHollandaiseSauce**
- Pinch paprika
- Pinch sea salt
- Pinch cayenne pepper
- 2 large free-range egg yolks
- 2 tablespoons of Ghee, melted
- 1 teaspoon freshly squeezed Meyer lemon juice
- ➢ **ForTheEggsBenedict**
- ½ cup Spiced Pulled Pork
- 1 teaspoon white vinegar
- 2 large free-range eggs

Instruction:

> **How to make the HollandaiseSauce**

1. Get a small bowl and gently whisk the egg yolks with the ghee, paprika, salt, lemon juice, and cayenne pepper.
2. Microwave the mixture for 20 seconds then whisk again until the sauce is smooth.

> **How to make the Eggs Benedict**

1. Get a small pot with water and let it boil.
2. Add the vinegar to the hot water.
3. Crack the eggs into a small bowl and roll around lightly.
4. Pour the eggs into the boiling water and poach for 3 minutes.
5. Meanwhile, get a plate and put the heated pulled pork.
6. Remove the poached eggs from the water anddry them.
7. Put the eggs on top of the pulled pork and put hollandaise sauce on them.
8. Serve immediately and enjoy!

OMELET WITH ASPARAGUS

Serving: 2

Prep Time: 10 Min

Cook Time: 20 Min

Ingredients:

- 1 cup shaved organic Havarti cheese
- 2 tablespoons chopped fresh thyme leaves
- 2 tablespoons chopped spring onions
- 1 tablespoon chopped wild fennel
- 1 cup 1-inch asparagus pieces
- 3 large free-range eggs
- 3 tablespoons organic heavy cream
- ½ teaspoon sea salt
- 2 tablespoons Ghee

Instructions:

1. Set a steamer rack inside a large pot and pour in enough water.
2. Let the water boil then add the asparagus.
3. Steam the asparagus until tender.
4. Drain the asparagus and set aside.

5. In a small bowl, beat together the eggs, heavy cream, and salt.

6. In a medium pan, melt the ghee over medium heat.

7. Pour the egg mixture into the pan and let it cook until it can be flipped without breaking.

8. Once the omelet is flipped, layer the cheese, thyme, onions,asparagus, and fennel over half of the omelet.

9. Continue cooking for 5 minutes more or until the cheese melts.

10. Fold the empty half of the omeletto the other half andput it in a plate.

11. Serve immediately.

FLUFFY CINNAMON AND CREAM CHEESE EGGS

Serving:6

PrepTime: 10 Min

Cook Time: 5 Min

Ingredients:

- ½ teaspoon ground cinnamon
- Sweetener
- 1 tablespoon Ghee
- Sugar-free maple syrup
- 6 tablespoons organic cream cheese, at room temperature
- 2 tablespoons organic heavy whipping cream
- 3 large free-range eggs
- 1 teaspoon coconut flour

Instruction:

1. In a blender, combine the cream cheese, heavy cream, eggs, cinnamon, coconut flour and sweetener to taste.

2. In a medium pan, melt the ghee over medium heat. Pour in the cream cheese and egg mixture.

3. Gently stir the mixture to scramble for 5 minutes.

4. Transfer to a plate and sprinkle with your favorite sugar-free maple syrup.

5. Serve immediately.

BREAKFAST-STYLE TACOS

Serving: 2

Prep Time: 10 Min

CookTime: 25 Min

Ingredients:

- 2 cups shredded organic Mexican cheese blend, divided
- 1 tablespoon of Ghee
- 1 avocado, peeled, pitted, and sliced
- Cayenne pepper sauce
- 3 large free-range eggs
- 2 tablespoons organic heavy cream
- 1 tablespoon Taco Seasoning
- Extra-virgin olive oil

Instructions:

1. Beatthe eggs, heavy cream, and taco seasoning then set aside.
2. To make the taco shells,Get a pan and grease it with olive oilthen place it over medium heat.

3. Once the oil is hot, put ½ cup of cheese in the
   pan.
4. Cook the cheesefor 3 to 5 minutes or until it
   starts to look brown. Remove it from the pan
   and form it into a taco-shell shape.
5. Let it stand upside down to cool.
6. Repeat the process to create more taco shells.
7. Put the pan on a medium heat and add the
   ghee. Once the ghee melts, stir the egg
   mixture and add it to the pan. Stir the eggs until
   scrambled.
8. Divide the eggs on the taco shells and top with
   avocado slices and cayenne pepper sauce.
9. Serve immediately and enjoy!

CHICKEN

RECIPES

BUFFALO CHICKEN BALLS WITH BLUE CHEESE

Serving: 4 to 6

PrepTime: 10 Min

CookTime: 18 Min

Ingredients:

- 2 tablespoons water
- 1 teaspoon onion powder
- ½ teaspoon sea salt
- ½ teaspoon freshly ground black pepper
- 1 recipe Buffalo Sauce
- 1 pound free-range ground chicken
- 1 large free-range egg
- 1 cup shredded organic mozzarella cheese
- ½ cup crumbled organic blue cheese
- ¼ cup chopped celery

Instructions:

1. Preheat the oven to 450°F.
2. Prepare a baking pan with parchment paper.

3. Get a large bowl, combine the chicken, egg, mozzarella and blue cheeses, celery, salt, pepper, water, and onion powder. Mix them all together.

4. Form the mixture into about 20 meatballs and place them on the baking pan.

5. Bake until the temperature reaches 165°F for15 minutes.

6. Meanwhile, warm the buffalo sauce in a saucepan over low heat.

7. When the meatballs are done, mix them in the warm sauce and serve.

CHICKEN CURRY WITH PUMPKIN

Serving: 2

Prep Time: 10 Min

CookTime: 15 Min

Ingredients:

- ½ teaspoon ground cinnamon
- ½ teaspoon ground ginger
- ½ teaspoon sea salt, plus additional for seasoning
- ½ teaspoon red pepper flakes
- 2 tablespoons extra-virgin olive oil
- 1 pound free-range chicken tenders
- Freshly ground black pepper
- 7 ounces pure pumpkin purée
- ½ cup unsweetened coconut milk
- 2 tablespoons Ghee
- 1 tablespoon freshly squeezed lime juice
- ½ small white onion, chopped
- 2 tablespoons chopped fresh Thai basil leaves

- 1 teaspoon curry powder
- ½ teaspoon ground coriander

Instructions:

1. In a blender, combine the pumpkin, coconut milk, ghee, lime juice, onion, Thai basil, cinnamon, ginger, curry powder, coriander salt, and red pepper flakes. Pour the mixture into a saucepan and set over medium heat.
2. In a medium pan, heat the olive oil over medium heat then season the chicken tenders with salt and black pepper.
3. When the oil is hot, cook the chicken tenders for about 3 minutes per side.
4. Cut the chicken to 1-inch pieces and add them to the pumpkin curry.
5. Reduce the heat and cook for 5 to 10 minutes more.
6. Serve hot and enjoy!

CHICKEN CORDON BLEU

Serving: 2

Prep Time: 10 Min

CookTime: 50 Min

Ingredients:

- ¼ cup shredded organic Appenzeller cheese
- ½ cup shredded organic Gruyère cheese
- ½ cup shredded organic Emmentaler cheese
- ⅛ teaspoon ground nutmeg
- ½ cup grated organic Parmesan cheese
- ½ teaspoon Seasoned Salt
- 2 large boneless, skinless
- 4 slices nitrate-free ham
- 2 teaspoons Dijon mustard
- 1 tablespoon extra-virgin olive oil

Instructions:

1. Preheat the oven to 375°F.
2. Prepare a rimmed baking sheet with parchment paper.

3. In a small bowl, combine the Emmentaler, Gruyère, and Appenzeller cheeses with the nutmeg.
4. Lay the chicken breasts flat on a surface and divide the cheese mixture between the two chicken breasts.
5. Place 2 slices of ham on top of the cheese on each chicken breast, then 1 teaspoon of Dijon mustard in the middle. Fold the chicken breast over to enclose the filling.
6. Brush the chicken with olive oil then sprinkle it withseasoned salt and Parmesan cheese.
7. Place the stuffed chicken breasts on the baking sheet and bake until the temperature reaches at least 165°F for 50 minutes.
8. Serve hot and enjoy!

MOZZARELLA-STUFFED CHICKEN CAPRESE

Serving: 2
Prep Time: 10 Min
CookTime: 40 Min

Ingredients:

- Sea salt
- 1 cup Roasted Red Peppers
- 2 tablespoons Italian seasoning
- Freshly ground black pepper
- 2 tablespoons extra-virgin olive oil
- 2 boneless chicken breasts,butterflied
- 10 fresh basil leaves
- 1 ball fresh organic mozzarella cheese, cut into 4 pieces

Ingredients:

1. Preheat the oven to 400°F.
2. Prepare a rimmed baking sheet with parchment paper.

3. Place five basil leaves inside each chicken
    breast.
4. Place two mozzarella slices inside each breast.
5. Divide the roasted red peppers between the
    two chicken breasts then sprinkle the Italian
    seasoning over each chicken breast and
    season them with salt and pepper. Close each
    chicken breast to envelop the filling.
6. Place the chicken breasts on the baking sheet
    and bake for 40 minutes.
7. Serve hot and enjoy!

LEMON AND GARLIC CHICKEN WITH CARAMELIZED ONIONS

Serving: 2

PrepTime: 10 Min and 1 HourtoMarinate

CookTime: 65 min

Ingredients:

- ¼ teaspoon paprika
- ⅛ teaspoon red pepper flakes
- 2 large boneless chicken breasts, butterflied
- 3 tablespoons freshly squeezed lemon juice
- 2 tablespoons minced garlic
- 1 teaspoon sea salt, plus additional for seasoning
- ¼ teaspoon freshly ground black pepper
- 1 yellow onion, quartered
- 2 cups trimmed green beans
- ¼ cup Ghee, melted
- 3 tablespoons extra-virgin olive oil

Instructions:

1. In a bowl or ziplockplastic bag, mix the olive oil, paprika, lemon juice, garlic, salt, red pepper and black pepper flakes. Add the chicken then coat it with the marinade.
2. Cover the bowl or seal the bag and marinate the chicken in the refrigerator for at least an hour.
3. Preheat the oven to 350°F.
4. Dice one of the onion quarters then cut the remaining three quarters into large portions.
5. Spread the larger portionsof onion across the bottom of an ovenproof pan then add the green beans, and scatter the diced onion on top.
6. Top theonion and green beans with the ghee then put the marinated chicken breasts.
7. Season the dish with a sprinkle of salt.
8. Bake the chicken until its temperature reaches at least 165°F for about 65 minutes.
9. Serve immediately and enjoy!

PARMESAN CHICKEN AND ZOODLES

Serving: 4

Prep Time: 10 Min

Cook Time: 45 Min

Ingredients:

- 2 cups crushed pork rinds
- 1 cup grated organic Parmesan cheese
- 2 tablespoons Italian seasoning
- 4 boneless chicken breasts, butterflied
- 1 cup shredded organic mozzarella cheese
- 4 small to medium zucchini
- 2 tablespoons garlic-infused olive oil
- 1 teaspoon garlic salt
- 1 cup Rhode Island Red Marinara Sauce

Instructions:

1. Preheat the oven to 375°F.

2. Prepare a rimmed baking sheet with parchment paper and set a wire rack on the parchment.
3. Get a large bowl, combine the pork rinds, Italian seasoningand Parmesan cheese.
4. Putthe chicken breast in the bowl one at a time and shake it until the chicken breast is totally covered in breading then place each breaded chicken breast on the wire rack.
5. Sprinkle the mozzarella cheese on the top of each chicken breast.
6. Bake the chicken for 30 to 45 minutes.
7. Meanwhile, spiralize the zucchini or use a vegetable peeler to shave it.
8. Place the zoodles in a bowl and mix them with the garlic oil and garlic salt. Set aside.
9. When the chicken breasts are cooked, remove them from the oven and transfer to a plate.
10. Getpan, warm the seasoned zoodles over medium-high heat. Cook them for 1 to 2 minutes. Add the marinara and continue cooking for 1 more minute.
11. Plate the zoodles next to the chicken then serve immediately.

BLUE CHEESE BUFFALO CHICKEN SALAD

Serving: 2

PrepTime: 10 Min

CookTime: 30 Min

Ingredients:

- 2 boneless, skinless free-range chicken breasts
- 4 uncured center-cut bacon strips
- ¼ cup Buffalo Sauce
- 4 cups chopped romaine lettuce, divided
- ½ cup blue cheese dressing, divided
- ½ cup crumbled organic blue cheese, divided
- ¼ cup chopped red onion, divided

Ingredients:

1. Bring a large pot of water and boil over high heat.

2. Add the chicken breasts to the water, reduce the heat to low, and cook the breasts until the temperature reaches 180°F for 30 minutes.

3. Transfer the chicken to a bowl and let it cool for 10 minutes.

4. Meanwhile, fry the bacon strips in a pan over medium heat for 3 minutes per side then drain the bacon.

5. Mixthe chicken with the buffalo sauce.

6. Divide the lettuce on two bowls. Put the half of the pulled chicken for each, then half of theblue cheese crumbles andblue cheese dressing, and chopped red onion. Smash the bacon over the salads and serve.

SPINACH RICOTTA CRÊPES WITH CHICKEN

Serving: 2

Prep Time: 15 Min

CookTime: 25 Min

Ingredients:

- 2 large boneless, chicken breasts, butterflied
- 4 cups chopped fresh spinach
- ¾ cup organic ricotta cheese
- ⅓ cup grated organic Parmesan cheese
- ¼ cup mayonnaise
- 1 tablespoon minced garlic
- ¼ teaspoon sea salt
- Pinch freshly ground black pepper
- Pinch red pepper flakes
- Pinch nutmeg
- Seasoned Salt

Instructions:

1. Preheat the oven to 425°F.

2. Prepare a rimmed baking sheet with parchment paper.
3. In a large bowl, mix the spinach, ricotta and Parmesan cheeses, garlic, salt, black pepper, red pepper flakes, mayonnaise and nutmeg.
4. Lay the chicken breasts flat on a surface and divide the spinach mixture between the two chicken breasts. Roll up each chicken breast and place it on the baking sheet then sprinkle with seasoned salt.
5. Bake until the temperature reaches 165°F for 25 minutes.
6. Serve hot and enjoy!

BLACK PEPPER CHICKEN

Serving: 2

PrepTime: 10 Min and 30 Min to Marinate

CookTime: 25 Min

Ingredients:

- ½ cup organic chicken broth
- ½ cup sake
- 3 tablespoons gluten-free oyster sauce
- 1 teaspoon tamari
- 2 garlic cloves, minced
- 1 tablespoon Creole seasoning
- 1 teaspoon freshly ground black pepper
- 1 teaspoon chili powder
- 1 teaspoon ground ginger
- 1 pound free-range chicken tenders, cut into 1-inch pieces
- ½ red onion, sliced
- ½ red bell pepper, cut into strips

Instructions:

1. In a medium bowl, mix together the chicken broth, sake, oyster sauce, tamari, garlic, pepper, ginger, chili powder, and Creole seasoning.
2. Add the chicken, red bell pepper, onion, and mix to coat.
3. Cover the bowl and marinate the chicken in the refrigerator for 25-30 minutes.
4. Preheat the oven to 350°F.
5. Transfer the chicken and marinade to an ovenproof pan. Bake the chicken and mix everything for 25 minutes.

CHEESY CHICKEN PARMESAN MEATBALLS

Serving: 5

Prep Time: 10 Min

CookTime: 25 Min

Ingredients:

- 1 pound free-range ground chicken
- 1 large free-range egg, lightly beaten
- 1 cup freshly grated organic Parmesan cheese
- ¾ cup shredded organic mozzarella cheese
- ¼ cup organic cream cheese, at room temperature
- 2 tablespoons water
- 3 garlic cloves, minced
- 1 teaspoon onion powder
- ½ teaspoon Italian seasoning
- ½ teaspoon sea salt
- ½ teaspoon freshly ground black pepper
- 8 slices organic provolone cheese, cut into strips

Instructions:

1. Preheat the oven to 450°F.
2. Prepare a baking pan with parchment paper.
3. Get a large bowl, combine the egg, chicken, Parmesan and mozzarella cheeses, cream cheese, garlic, onion powder, Italian seasoning, salt, pepper, and water.
4. Mix the ingredients well.
5. Form the mixture into about 20 meatballs and place them in the baking pan.
6. Bake the meatballs until they reach atemperature of 165°F for20 minutes.
7. Remove the baking pan from the oven. Turn the oven to broil.
8. Place the strips of provolone on the meatballs then place them under the broiler for 3 to 5 minutes.
9. Serve immediately and enjoy!

PORK

RECIPES

MOZZARELLA STICKS WITH BACON

Serving: 3

PrepTime: 10 Min and 1 hourtofreeze

CookTime: 15 Min

Ingredients:

- 6 whole-milk organic mozzarella cheese sticks
- 12 uncured center-cut bacon strips

Instructions:

1. Prepare a rimmed baking sheet with parchment paper.
2. Place the cheese sticks on the sheet then freeze for 45mins to 1 hour.
3. Preheat the oven to 400°F.
4. Wrap each cheese stick in two strips of bacon then baked for 10-15minutes
5. Serve immediately and enjoy!

RED PEPPERS CHORIZO BOMBS

Serving: 4

Prep Time: 10 Min

CookTime: 40 Min

Ingredients:

- ½ teaspoon ground cumin
- ¼ teaspoon ground paprika
- ¼ cup roughly chopped fresh cilantro
- 1 cup shredded organic Cheddar cheese, divided
- 4 red bell peppers, tops cut off, seeds and membranes removed
- 1 tablespoon extra-virgin olive oil
- ¼ cup chopped onion
- 1 pound bulk Mexican chorizo
- ½ teaspoon freshly ground black pepper

Instructions:

1. Preheat the oven to 400°F.
2. Prepare a rimmed baking sheet with parchment paper.

3. Cut the red bell peppers side up and place them on the baking sheet.

4. Get apan, heat the olive oil over low heat then when it is hot, add the onion for 3 minutes.

5. Add the chorizo, paprika, black pepper, and cuminthen cook until the meat is browned. Continue cookingfor 5 minutes then stir in the cilantro.

6. Put the chorizo mixture into the red bell peppers.

7. Put ¼ cup of Cheddar cheese for each then bake for about 30 minutes.

8. Serve immediately and enjoy!

KALE CREAM SOUP

Serving: 4 to 6

Prep Time: 10 Min

CookTime: 20 Min

Ingredients:

- 1 tablespoon minced garlic
- ½ teaspoon red pepper flakes
- ½ teaspoon freshly ground black pepper
- ½ teaspoon Italian seasoning
- Sea salt
- 2 cups chopped kale
- 1 pound organic bulk Italian sausage
- ½ cup chopped pancetta
- ½ cup chopped onion
- 2 cups organic heavy cream
- 2 cups organic chicken broth

Instructions:

1. Get a large pot and sauté the Italian sausage, pancetta, and onion over a medium heat for 5 minutes.

2. Stir in the heavy cream, chicken broth, garlic, red pepper flakes, black pepper, and Italian seasoning. Boil the soup then reduce the heat to simmer.

3. Season the soup with salt and let it simmer for 10 minutes.

4. Add in the kale and simmer for 5 more minutes.

5. Serve immediately and enjoy!

LOW-CARB QUESADILLA WITH CHICKEN

Serving: 2

Prep Time: 10 Min

CookTime: 40 Min

Ingredients:

- ¼ cup ranch dressing
- ½ cup shredded organic Cheddar cheese
- 20 uncured center-cut bacon strips
- 2 cups sliced grilled free-range chicken

Instructions:

1. Preheat the oven to 400°F.
2. Prepare a rimmed baking sheet with parchment paper.
3. Lay out 5 bacon strips right next to each other on the sheet. Weave the 5 bacon strips into the first layer of the opposite direction to createa woven bacon square. Repeat this with the remaining bacon strips to make another woven bacon square.

4. Bake for 30 minutes.

5. Trim the bacon squares to have the same size and shape.

6. Layer the grilled chicken over one bacon square then drizzle it with the ranch dressing.

7. Sprinkle with the Cheddar cheese then top it with the second bacon square.

8. Discard the previous parchment paper and line the baking sheet with a new one.

9. Bake the quesadilla for 5 to 10 minutes or until the cheese melts.

10. Cut in half, serve, and enjoy!

BACON JERKY WITH BLACK PEPPER

Serving: 6

Prep Time: 10 Min

CookTime: 2 Hours

Ingredients:

- 1 tablespoon chili powder
- 1½ teaspoons freshly ground black pepper
- 1 pound uncured center-cut bacon
- 1 tablespoon garlic powder
- 1 tablespoon ground cumin
- 1 tablespoon smoked paprika

Instruction:

1. Preheat the oven between 150°F and 175°F.
2. Get a large bowl, mix the chili powder, paprika, garlic powder, cumin, and pepper. Add the strips of bacon to the bowl and coat them all over with the rub.

3. Place the baking sheets on the bottom rack of
    the oven to catch any fat that from the bacon.
4. Bake for at least 2 hours.
5. Remove the bacon once it reaches your
    desired jerkiness.
6. Serve immediately and enjoy!

SAGE MEATLOAF WITH ORANGE ZEST

Serving: 4
Prep Time: 15 Min
CookTime: 45 Min

Ingredients:

- 1 pound organic bulk sweet Italian sausage
- 2 cups crushed pork rinds
- 2 cups shredded organic mozzarella cheese
- 3 large free-range eggs, lightly beaten
- ⅓ cup organic heavy cream
- 2 tablespoons Worcestershire sauce
- ½ yellow onion, chopped
- 4 large fresh sage leaves, chopped
- ½ teaspoon garlic powder
- ½ teaspoon onion powder
- 1 teaspoon sea salt
- ½ teaspoon freshly ground black pepper
- 2 tablespoons grated orange zest

Instructions:

1. Preheat the oven to 350°F.

2. In a large bowl, combine the sausage, pork rinds, heavy cream, worcestershire sauce, onion, sage, mozzarella cheese, eggs, garlic powder, onion powder, pepper,and salt. Mixall the ingredients then evenly pack the meatloaf mixture into a baking dish. After that, sprinkle the orange zest on the top of the meat.

3. Bake for 45 minutes. Let sit for 5 minutes, then slice and serve.

PORK CHOPS WITH WALNUT CRUST

Serving: 2

Prep Time: 10 Min

CookTime: 20 Min

Ingedients:

- Pinch freshly ground black pepper
- 1 large free-range egg
- 2 boneless free-range pork chops
- 3 tablespoons crushed walnuts
- 3 tablespoons grated organic Parmesan cheese
- Pinch sea salt

Instructions

1. Preheat the oven to 400°F.
2. Prepare a rimmed baking sheet with parchment paper.
3. In a bowl, mix the walnuts, Parmesan cheese, salt, and pepper.

4. In medium-bowl, beat the egg.

5. Dip the pork chops in the egg, coat it with the Parmesan mixture, walnut, and place it on the baking sheet.

6. Bake the pork chops for 10-12 minutes, flip them and bake them again for another 10-12 minutes.

7. Serve immediately and enjoy!

ROASTED PORK CHOPS WITH GARLIC GREEN BEANS

Serving: 4

Prep Time: 10 Min

CookTime: 30 Min

Ingredients:

- ½ teaspoon garlic salt
- 5 fresh thyme sprigs
- ½ cup grated organic Parmesan cheese
- ½ cup freshly shaved organic Parmesan cheese
- 4 tablespoons garlic-infused olive oil, divided
- 4 thick-cut boneless free-range pork chops
- 2 cups trimmed green beans
- 10 garlic cloves, peeled

Instructions:

1. Preheat the oven to 350°F.
2. Get an ovenproof pan, put 2 tablespoons of garlic-infused olive oil to coat the bottom. Add

the pork chops, then in between the porkchops and around the edges, distribute the garlic cloves and the green beans.

3. Put the remaining oil over the top of the meat and vegetables.

4. Sprinkle with the garlic salt then place the thyme sprigs on top. Lastly, sprinkle with the grated Parmesan cheese.

5. Bake for 30 minutes.

6. Serve immediately and enjoy!

SPICY PULLED PORK

Serving: 10

Prep Time: 10 Min

Cook Time: 8 to 12 Hours

Ingredients:

- 1 tablespoon garlic powder
- 1 tablespoon sea salt
- 1 teaspoon ground mustard
- 1 teaspoon cayenne pepper
- ½ cup organic chicken broth
- 3 drops liquid smoke
- ½ onion, sliced
- 1 free-range pork butt
- 1 tablespoon paprika
- 1 tablespoon chili powder
- 1 tablespoon onion powder

Instructions:

1. Set your slow cooker to low then pour in the liquid smoke and the broth then add the onion slices. Place the pork butt on the sliced onions.

2. In a small bowl, mix the paprika, onion powder, garlic powder, salt, ground mustard, cayenne pepper, and ,chilli powder then rub the mixture on the pork butt.

3. Cover and cook for 8 to 10 hours.

4. Transfer the pork to a large plate and use two forks to pull it apart.

5. Get a blender, purée the juices and onions from the slow cooker.

6. Mix the sauce into the pulled pork, serve, and enjoy!

PORK FLORENTINE WITH LEMON-CAPER SAUCE

Serving: 2 to 4

Prep Time: 10 Min

CookTime: 30 Min

Ingredients:

- 2 garlic cloves, minced
- 4 teaspoons freshly squeezed lemon juice
- 4 teaspoons grated lemon zest
- 2 teaspoons chopped fresh parsley
- 20 spinach leaves
- 8 boneless free-range pork cutlets
- 2 tablespoons drained capers
- ½ cup salted grass-fed butter
- 2 tablespoons chopped sweet white onion

Instructions:

1. Preheat the oven to 375°F.

2. In a baking dish, layer the spinach leaves
    between the pork cutlets and scatter the
    capers to the pork and spinach.
3. In a saucepan, melt the butter over low heat.
    Add the garlic and onion, cook until soft then
    stir the butter for 2 minutes more.
4. Whisk in the lemon juice and zest and the
    parsley then pour the sauce over the pork
    cutlets.
5. Bake for 25 minutes.
6. Serve hot and enjoy!

BEEF &LAMB RECIPES

BAKED ITALIAN MEATBALLS

Serving: 5

Prep Time: 20 Min

CookTime: 20 Min

Ingredients:

- 1 tablespoon minced garlic
- 1 tablespoon Italian seasoning
- 1 teaspoon Cajun seasoning
- 1 teaspoon sea salt
- 1 teaspoon freshly ground black pepper
- 1 ball fresh organic mozzarella cheese
- 1 pound grass-fed ground beef
- 1 pound free-range ground pork
- 1 large free-range egg, lightly beaten
- 1 tablespoon water
- ½ cup shredded organic mozzarella cheese
- ½ cup freshly grated organic Parmesan cheese

Instructions:

1. Preheat the oven to 400°F.

2. Prepare a rimmed baking sheet with
    parchment paper.
3. Get a large bowl, combine the beef, pork, egg,
    water, mozzarella, salt, pepper, Parmesan
    cheeses, garlic, Cajun seasoning, and Italian
    seasoning. Mix thoroughly and form the
    mixture into meatballs of your preferred size.
4. Cut the mozzarella into cubes then stuff a one
    into each meatball. After that, place each
    stuffed meatball on the baking sheet.
5. Bake the meatballs for 20 minutes.
6. Serve hot and enjoy!

LOW-CARB MEATZZA

Serving: 2 to 3

Prep Time: 10 Min

CookTime: 30 Min

Ingredients:

- 1 teaspoon fennel seed
- ½ cup Rhode Island Red Marinara Sauce
- 1 cup shredded organic mozzarella cheese
- ¼ cup chopped green bell pepper
- ¼ cup chopped red onion
- Grass-fed butter, at room temperature
- 8 ounces grass-fed ground beef
- 8 ounces free-range ground pork
- ½ cup grated organic Parmesan cheese
- 2 tablespoons water
- 1½ teaspoons pizza seasoning

Instructions:

1. Preheat the oven to 400°F.
2. Butter a pie dish.

3. In a large-size bowl, mix the beef, pork, pizza seasoning, fennel, Parmesan cheese, and water. Flatten out the mixture on the bottom of the pie dish.

4. Bake for 15 to 20 minutes or until the meat has browned.

5. Top the meat crust with marinara, onion, mozzarella cheese, and green bell pepper.

6. Bake for another 10 minutes

7. Slice, serve, and enjoy!

SWEDISH MEATBALLS

Serving: 4

Prep Time: 10 Min

CookTime: 2½ Hours

Ingredients:

- 4 tablespoons salted grass-fed butter
- 1½ cups organic chicken broth
- 1½ cups organic heavy cream
- 1 tablespoon Dijon mustard
- 1 tablespoon Worcestershire sauce
- 1 pound grass-fed ground beef
- 1 pound free-range ground pork
- 1 cup shredded mild organic Cheddar cheese
- 1 large free-range egg
- 1 tablespoon water
- ¼ cup diced onion
- ¼ teaspoon ground nutmeg
- ¼ teaspoon ground allspice

Instructions:

1. Preheat the oven to 400°F.

2. Prepare a large baking pan with parchment paper.

3. In a large-size bowl, combine the beef, pork, onion, nutmeg, allspice, Cheddar cheese, egg, and water. Roll the mixture into your preferred size of the meatballs and put them in the lined baking pan.

4. Bake for 20 minutes.

5. Meanwhile, in another pan, heat the butter, heavy cream and chicken broth, over medium heat. Once it simmer, reduce the heat to low and let it simmer again for 20 minutes or until it reduces to half then add in the Worcestershire sauce and mustard.

6. Pour the sauce and add the meatballs when they're ready.

7. Cook on low for 2 hours.

8. Serve immediately and enjoy!

BEEF FONDUE WITH GARLIC AND THYME

Serving: 4 to 6

Prep Time: 10 Min

CookTime: 10 Min

Ingrdients:

- 1 tablespoon sea salt
- 1 tablespoon freshly ground black pepper
- 3 fresh thyme sprigs
- Thin slices of grass-fed beef filet and
- 4 cups organic beef broth
- 1 cup dry red wine
- 1 shallot, chopped
- 2 tablespoons minced garlic

Instructions:

1. Set the fondue pot on high then combine the shallot, garlic, salt, pepper, thyme, beef broth, and red wine.
2. Let it simmer.

3. Use your fondue forks to cook single pieces of meat at a time. Each piece of meat will take 1 to 3 minutes to reach your preferred doneness.

STIR-FRY BEEF

Serving: 4

PrepTime: 10 Min

CookTime: 10 Min

Ingredients:

- ⅛ teaspoon ground ginger
- 1 cup pea pods, trimmed
- ¼ cup chopped broccoli
- 1 scallion, chopped
- 1 pound grass-fed ground beef
- 3 large free-range eggs
- 1 tablespoon tamari
- 1 tablespoon peanut butter

Instructions:

1. In a pan, cook the ground beef over medium-high heat for 3 minutes.
2. Remove the beef from the pan, then crack and scramble the eggs for 1 minute.

3. Return the meat to the pan and add in the
    ginger, pea pods, broccoli, scallion, tamari, and
    peanut butter.
4. Cover and cook for 5 minutes.
5. Serve and enjoy!

BAKED BACON-WRAPPED MEATBALLS

Serving: 6

PrepTime: 20 Min

CookTime: 30 Min

Ingredients:

- 2 teaspoons freshly ground black pepper
- 1 tablespoon Italian seasoning
- 2 or 3 onions
- 1 pound uncured center-cut bacon
- 1 pound grass-fed ground beef
- 1 pound free-range ground pork
- 2 large free-range eggs, lightly beaten
- 1 cup grated organic Parmesan cheese
- 1 cup shredded organic mozzarella cheese
- ¾ cup minced garlic or garlic paste

Instructions:

1. Preheat the oven to 350°F.

2. Prepare a rimmed baking sheet with parchment paper.

3. Get a large bowl, combine the beef, pork, eggs, garlic, pepper, Italian seasoning,Parmesan, and mozzarella cheeses. Mix the ingredients well and form large meatballs.

4. Cut the top and bottom off each onion and separate its layers. Stuff each onion shell with a meatball.

5. Wrap each onion ball with bacon then place each wrapped meatball on the baking sheet.

6. Bake the meatballs for 30 minutes.

7. Serve hot and enjoy!

CHILI-CRUSTED NEW YORK STRIPS

Serving: 4
PrepTime: 5 Min
CookTime: 10 Min

Ingredients:

- 1 teaspoon freshly ground black pepper
- ⅛ teaspoon chili powder
- 2 grass-fed New York strip steaks
- ¼ cup Ghee, melted
- 1 teaspoon minced garlic
- Leaves from 2 rosemary sprigs
- 2 teaspoons sea salt

Instructions:

1. Get a bowl, combine the salt, pepper, ghee, garlic, rosemary, and chili powder then rub the mixture into both steaks.
2. In a pan, sear the steaks over medium heat on each side for 3-5 minutes per side.

3. Plate the steaks and let them rest for 3-5
    minutes.
4. Serve hot and enjoy!

LOW-CARB PHILLY CHEESESTEAK MEATLOAF

Serving: 4

PrepTime: 10 Min

CookTime: 45 Min

Ingredients:

- 1 teaspoon sea salt
- ½ teaspoon freshly ground black pepper
- ½ teaspoon garlic powder
- ½ teaspoon onion powder
- 4 cups shredded organic American cheese, divided
- 1 pound grass-fed ground beef
- ½ yellow onion, chopped
- 1 green bell pepper, seeded and chopped
- ⅓ cup organic heavy cream
- 2 tablespoons Worcestershire sauce

Instructions:

1. Preheat the oven to 350°F.

2. In a large bowl, mix the beef, onion, green bell
    pepper, heavy cream, pepper, garlic powder,
    onion powder Worcestershire sauce, and salt.
3. Spread half of the mixture in the bottom of a
    baking dish. Put 2 cups of American cheese
    then layer the remaining meatloaf on top of the
    cheese.
4. Bake for 45 minutes then let it rest for 5
    minutes.
5. Slice, serve, and enjoy!

MEXICAN CASSEROLE

Serving: 6

Prep Time: 10 Min

CookTime: 20 Min

Ingredients:

- ¼ cup water
- ¼ cup Taco Seasoning
- 2 cups organic sour cream
- 2 cups shredded lettuce
- 2 cups shredded organic Cheddar cheese
- Cayenne pepper sauce
- 2 ripe avocados, peeled, pitted, and cut into chunks
- 1 tablespoon freshly squeezed lime juice
- ¼ cup chopped fresh cilantro
- ¼ cup diced white onion
- 1 tomato, seeded and chopped
- 1 teaspoon minced garlic
- ½ teaspoon sea salt
- 2 pounds grass-fed ground beef

Instructions:

1. In a bowl, mash together the cilantro, onion, tomato, avocado, lime juice, garlic, and salt. Cover the guacamole and refrigerate while you make the rest of the casserole.
2. In a medium pan, cook the ground beef over medium heat for 10 minutes.
3. Add in water and taco seasoning.
4. Reduce the heat to simmer and cook for 10 minutes.
5. Transfer the meat to a plate, top it with the sour cream, and then top again with guacamole.
6. Sprinkle the lettuce over the guacamole and top it with Cheddar cheese.
7. Drizzle on some cayenne pepper sauce then serve, and enjoy!

FISH &

SHELLFISH

RECIPES

COFFEE-RUBBED TUNA STEAK

Serving: 2

PrepTime: 5 min and 30 minto rest

CookTime: 5 min

Ingredients:

- 1 teaspoon sea salt
- ½ teaspoon ground cinnamon
- ½ teaspoon chili powder
- 2 high-quality tuna steaks
- Extra-virgin olive oil
- 3 tablespoons finely ground coffee
- 1 tablespoon freshly ground black pepper

Instructions:

1. Using olive oil, brush all tuna steaks.
2. In a small bowl, combine the chili powder, coffee, pepper, salt, and cinnamon.
3. Sprinkle the coffee mixture on both sides of the steaks and let them rest.
4. In a medium pan, sear the tuna on both sides on a high heat until you forma crust.

5. Serve hot and enjoy!

SPICY SALMON FLORENTINE

Serving: 2

Prep Time: 10 Min

Cook Time: 25 Min

Ingredients:

- 3 sun-dried tomatoes, chopped
- 4 thin-cut boneless, skinless salmon fillets
- Fresh spinach leaves
- Sea salt
- Freshly ground black pepper
- 2 lemon quarters, for garnish
- ½ cup organic cream cheese, at room temperature
- ¼ cup organic ricotta cheese
- ¼ teaspoon red pepper flakes
- 1 tablespoon Ghee
- ¼ cup minced shallot
- 2 garlic cloves, minced

Instructions:

1. Preheat the oven to 350°F.

2. Prepare a rimmed baking sheet with parchment paper.
3. In a bowl, mix thered pepper flakes, cream cheese, and ricotta cheese then set aside.
4. In a pan, melt the ghee on a medium heat then add the sun-dried tomatoes, shallot and garlic.
5. Cook for 3 to 5 minutes.
6. Add the shallot mixture into the cheese mixture.
7. Lay out 2 salmon fillets on the baking sheet.
8. Spread half of the cheese mixture on the 2 fillets.
9. Put spinach leaves on top of the cheese.
10. Put the remaining salmon fillets on top of the cheese.
11. Season with black pepper and salt.
12. Bake the salmon for 15 to 20 minutes.
13. Serve hot and enjoy!

SALMON WITH GARLIC AND THYME

Serving: 2 to 4

Prep Time: 10 Min

CookTime: 10 Min

Ingredients:

- 4 salmon fillets
- 1 onion, quartered
- ¼ lemon
- 4 tablespoons Ghee, divided
- 1 tablespoon minced garlic
- 1 tablespoon fresh thyme leaves
- Pinch sea salt

Instructions:

1. Preheat the oven to 450°F.
2. In a bowl, pour 2 tablespoons of ghee and mix it with garlic, thyme, and salt then set aside.
3. In a medium pan, melt the remaining ghee over medium heat.

4. Add the salmon fillets then wedge the onion
   quarters between each fillet.
5. Sear the salmon fillets for 1 minute then flip
   and sear for another minute.
6. Break the onion quarters into separate layers
   then top the salmon with the seasoning
   mixture.
7. Bake for 8 to 10 minutes.
8. Serve hot and enjoy!

BAKED HADDOCK WITHSAGE AND SAUSAGE

Serving: 4

Prep Time: 10 Min

CookTime: 45 Min

Ingredients:

- Sea salt
- Freshly ground black pepper
- 2 tablespoons freshly squeezed lemon juice, divided
- 1 tablespoon grated lemon zest
- 1 tablespoon minced garlic
- 4 haddock fillets
- 1 pound organic bulk sausage
- 2 tablespoons chopped fresh sage
- 1 cup thinly sliced fennel
- 10 cherry tomatoes, halved
- 1 onion, quartered
- 2 teaspoons garlic-infused olive oil

Instructions:

1. Preheat the oven to 400°F.

2. In an ovenproof pan, cook the sage and
    sausage on a medium-high heat for 5 minutes
    or until the meat is browned.

3. Remove the meat from the pan and set aside.

4. Add the fennel to the pan and top it with
    theonion quarters and tomatoes.

5. Put the garlic olive oil over the top.

6. Season with salt and pepper then drizzle some
    lemon juice over the vegetables.

7. Place the pan in the oven for 30 minutes while
    stirring the vegetables once in a while.

8. Meanwhile, in a bowl, mix the remainingminced
    garlic, lemon juice, and lemon zest.

9. Put the fillets in the mixture then set aside.

10. Once the vegetables are roasted, add the
    sausage to the pan and mix well.

11. Place the fillets on top of the vegetable-
    sausage mix.

12. Bake the fillets for 10 minutes.

13. Serve hot and enjoy!

SPICY LOBSTER SALAD

Serving: 1

PrepTime: 10 Min

Ingredients:

- Pinch sea salt
- 1 cup frozen precooked Maine lobster meat
- ¼ cup chopped celery
- ⅓ cup mayonnaise
- 1 tablespoon freshly squeezed lemon juice
- 1 teaspoon sriracha
- 1½ teaspoons minced fresh tarragon

Instructions:

1. In a bowl, mix the mayonnaise,sriracha, tarragon, lemon juice, and salt.
2. Stir in the lobster and celery then mix well.
3. Serve and enjoy!

CREAMY SEAFOOD CHOWDER

Serving: 6

Prep Time: 10 Min

CookTime: 1 Hour

Ingredients:

- 1 bay leaf
- 1 pound minced clams
- 1 pound frozen precooked langostinos
- 1 cup organic heavy cream
- 3 dashes Worcestershire sauce
- ½ teaspoon sea salt
- 1 teaspoon freshly ground black pepper
- 3 tablespoons Ghee
- 1 ounce salt pork
- ½ white onion, diced
- 1 teaspoon minced garlic
- 1½ cups clam juice
- 1 cup organic chicken broth
- ½ teaspoon celery salt
- ½ teaspoon dried tarragon

- ¼ teaspoon dried thyme

Instructions:

1. In a medium saucepan, melt the ghee on a medium heat. Add the garlic, pork, and onion and cook for 5 minutes.
2. Add the broth, clam juice, bay leafcelery salt, tarragon, and thyme. Reduce the heat to medium-low and let it simmer for 30 minutes.
3. Add the langostinosand clams to the pot then increase the heatuntil it boil. After that, reduce the heat to low and then simmer the soup for 5 to 10 minutes.
4. Add in the Worcestershire sauce, heavy cream, salt, and pepper.
5. Simmer for another 10 minutes.
6. Serve hot and enjoy!

LEMON BUTTER BAKED COD

Serving: 2

Prep Time: 10 Min

CookTime: 20 Min

Ingredients:

- 4 tablespoons salted grass-fed butter, divided
- 4 fresh thyme sprigs, divided
- 4 teaspoons freshly squeezed lemon juice, divided
- 4 cod fillets, rinsed and patted dry
- Sea salt
- Freshly ground black pepper

Instructions:

1. Preheat the oven to 400°F.
2. Season the fillets with salt and pepper on both sides.
3. Lay out an aluminum foil.
4. Place the fillet in the center of each piece of foil.

5. Divide the lemon juice, butter, and thyme among all fillets.

6. Fold the sides of each foil sheet to form a pouch to seal the fillet inside.

7. Place all foil pouches on a rimmed baking sheet.

8. Bake for 20 minutes.

9. Serve hot and enjoy!

BACON-WRAPPED TILAPIA

Serving: 2 to 4

PrepTime: 10 Min

CookTime: 30 Min

Ingredients:

- Freshly ground black pepper
- 12 uncured center-cut bacon strips
- ¼ cup mayonnaise
- 1½ tablespoons freshly squeezed lemon juice
- 4 tilapia fillets, rinsed and patted dry
- 3 tablespoons Ghee, melted
- 1 teaspoon dried basil

Instructions:

1. Preheat the oven to 375°F.
2. Prepare a rimmed baking sheet with parchment paper.
3. Brush all the fillets with the ghee then sprinkle them with few grinds of pepper andbasil.
4. Wrap three to four slices of bacon around each tilapia fillet and place them on the baking sheet.

5. Bake the filletsfor 20 to 30 minutes.

6. In a small bowl, whisk together the lemon juice, mayonnaise, and a pinch of pepper.

7. Serve hot and enjoy!

LEMON AND PARMESAN FISH STICKS

Serving: 2

Prep Time: 10 Min

CookTime: 15 Min

Ingredients:

- 1 tablespoon almond flour
- 1 teaspoon lemon pepper seasoning or Cajun seasoning
- Extra-virgin olive oil
- 1 large free-range egg
- ½ cup crushed pork rinds, crushed fine in a blender
- ¼ cup grated organic Parmesan cheese
- 4 tilapia or cod fillets, rinsed, patted dry, and cut into 1-by-4-inch strips

Instructions:

1. Preheat the oven to 400°F.

2. Prepare a rimmed baking sheet with aluminum
    foil. Place a wire rack over the baking sheet
    and lightly grease it with a little olive oil.
3. In a bowl, lightly beat the egg.
4. In another bowl, combine the Parmesan
    cheese, almond flour, crushed pork rinds, and
    lemon pepper seasoning.
5. Dip each strip into the beaten egg, thendip on
    dry mix. Place each strip on the rack over the
    baking sheet.
6. Bake the fish sticks for 15 minutes.
7. Serve hot and enjoy!

GARLIC SHRIMP

Serving: 2

PrepTime: 10 Min

CookTime: 10 Min

Ingredients:

- Pinch sea salt
- Pinch freshly ground black pepper
- 1 tablespoon organic Parmesan cheese
- 2 tablespoons Ghee
- 2 garlic cloves, minced
- 20 medium shrimp, peeled and deveined
- Pinch red pepper flakes

Instructions:

1. In a pan, melt the ghee on a medium-high heat.
2. Add the garlic and cook for 1 to 2 minutes.
3. Then add the shrimp and cook for 2 minutes.
4. Stir in the salt, pepper, and red pepper flakes,.
5. Sauté the shrimp for 5 more minutes.

6. Add in the Parmesan cheese, serve, and
    enjoy!

ZOODLES, SALADS, & SIDE DISHES RECIPES

AGLIO E OLIO ZOODLES

Serving: 1

PrepTime: 10 Min

CookTime: 3 Min

Ingredients:

- Sea salt
- Freshly ground black pepper
- 1 tablespoon grated organic Parmesan cheese
- Pinch chopped fresh parsley
- 2 tablespoons Ghee
- 1 tablespoon minced garlic
- Pinch red pepper flakes
- 2 heaping cups spiralized zucchini

Instructions:

1. In a medium saucepan, melt the ghee on a medium heat then add the garlic and red pepper flakes. Cook for 1 minute.
2. Add the zucchini and stir. Continue cooking for 1 to 2 minutes.

3. Season with the salt and black pepper then
    toss with the Parmesan cheese and parsley.
4. Serve immediately and enjoy!

LEMON-RICOTTA ZOODLES

Serving: 2

PrepTime: 10 Min

CookTime: 5 Min

Ingredients:

- 4 chard leaves, stemmed and chopped
- ½ shallot, minced
- 2 heaping cups spiralized zucchini
- 1½ teaspoons fresh thyme leaves
- ½ cup organic ricotta cheese
- Grated zest of 1 lemon
- Pinch sea salt
- Pinch freshly ground black pepper
- 1 tablespoon Ghee

Instructions:

1. In a bowl, mix the pepper, ricotta cheese, zest, and salt then set aside.
2. In a large pan, melt the ghee on a medium heat then add the chard and sauté for 1 to 2 minutes.

3. Add the shallot and sauté for another minute.
4. Add in the zucchini noodles and thyme and cook for 1 minute.
5. Add in the ricotta mixture and cook for another 2 minutes.
6. Serve immediately and enjoy!

BACON AND BLUE CHEESE ZOODLES

Serving: 1
Prep Time: 10 Min

Ingredients:

- ½ cup cooked and crumbled uncured center-cut bacon
- Freshly cracked black pepper
- 1 cup spiralized zucchini
- ½ cup baby spinach
- 3 tablespoons chunky blue cheese dressing
- ⅓ cup crumbled organic blue cheese

Instructions:

1. In a bowl, mix together the zucchini, blue cheese, bacon, spinach, dressing and pepper.
2. Serve cold.

CHICKEN PAD THAI

Serving: 4

Prep Time: 20 Min

CookTime: 10 Min

Ingredients:

- 2 tablespoons tamari
- 1 tablespoon rice vinegar
- ½ cup chopped scallion
- 2 garlic cloves, minced
- 1 teaspoon red pepper flakes
- 4 zucchini, spiralized
- ½ cup bean sprouts
- ½ cup crushed peanuts, for garnish
- 1 lime, cut into wedges, for garnish
- ⅛ teaspoon ground ginger
- ⅛ teaspoon garlic powder
- ⅛ teaspoon sea salt
- ⅛ teaspoon freshly ground black pepper
- 2 pounds free-range chicken tenders
- 2 tablespoons peanut oil

- 3 large free-range eggs, lightly beaten
- ⅓ cup organic chicken broth
- 3 tablespoons peanut butter

Instructions:

1. Get a medium bowl, mix the salt, ginger, garlic powder, and black pepper.
2. Add the chicken tenders.
3. In a pan, heat the peanut oil on a medium-high heat then add the chicken tenders and cook for 3 minutes.
4. Remove the chicken from the pan and cut into thick slices then set aside.
5. Add the eggs to the pan and scramble for 1 minute. Once cooked, remove from the pan and set aside.
6. Reduce the heat to medium-low and add the scallion, garlic, chicken broth, peanut butter, tamari, vinegar, and red pepper flakes. Stir and cook for 3 minutes.
7. Add the chicken slices, zucchini noodles, scrambled eggs, and sprouts to the pan and cook for 1 minute.
8. Serve hot and enjoy!

TOMATO BURRATA CAPRESE SALAD

Serving: 2 to 4

PrepTime: 5 Min

Ingredients:

- 1 ball organic burrata cheese
- Extra-virgin olive oil
- Coarsely ground black pepper
- 2 medium tomatoes
- Sea salt
- 10 fresh basil leaves

Instructions:

1. Slice the tomatoes and sprinkle with salt then put them on a plate.
2. Chop the basil leaves and sprinkle them on top of the tomato slices.
3. Add the burrata ball to the top then season with salt and pepper.
4. Slice the burrata to serve. Enjoy!

ROASTED GARLIC

Serving: 4

Prep Time: 10 Min

CookTime: 1 Hour

Ingredients:

- 1 teaspoon fresh thyme leaves
- 1 head elephant garlic
- 1 tablespoon Ghee

Instructions:

1. Preheat the oven to 400°F.
2. Cut off the top of the garlic to expose most of the cloves.
3. Place the head of the garlic on a sheet of aluminum foil then add the ghee to the top of the cloves and sprinkle with the salt and thyme.
4. Wrap the head loosely in the foil and place it in the baking dish.
5. Bake for 1 hour.
6. Use a fork to pluck each clove.
7. Serve as isand enjoy!

SPICY BUTTERED BEANS

Serving: 4

Prep Time: 5 Min

CookTime: 10 Min

Ingredients:

- Pinch red pepper flakes
- Pinch sea salt
- 4 cups trimmed green beans
- 2 tablespoons Ghee
- 2 garlic cloves, minced

Instructions:

1. Get a medium pot with water and salt then boil.
2. Add the green beans and cook for 3 minutes.
3. Meanwhile, prepare a bowl of ice water. Drain the green beans and drop them immediately into the ice water to stop them from cooking. Once cooled, drain the beans and set aside.
4. In a pan, melt the ghee over medium heat then add the garlic, red pepper flakes, and salt and cook for 1 minute.

5. Add the green beans and mix until hot for
    about 3 minutes

6. Serve immediately and enjoy!

LOW-CARB CAULIFLOWER RISOTTO

Serving: 4

Prep Time: 10 Min

CookTime: 6 Min

Ingredients:

- 1 tablespoon grated lemon zest
- 1 tablespoon freshly squeezed lemon juice
- ½ cup chopped fresh herbs, such as thyme, basil, rosemary, and/or sage
- 2 tablespoons shredded organic Parmesan cheese
- Florets from 1 head cauliflower
- 1 tablespoon minced shallot
- 2 tablespoons Ghee
- ⅓ cup organic mascarpone

Instructions:

1. Put the cauliflower florets in a food processor or blender. Pulse until the cauliflower looks like grains of rice.
2. In a large microwave-safe bowl, combine the cauliflower, ghee, and shallot.
3. Microwave for 5 minutes.
4. Add in the mascarpone and microwave for another minute.
5. Fold in the lemon zest, lemon juice, and herbs, and toss with the Parmesan cheese.
6. Serve hot and enjoy!

PESTO GNOCCHI

Serving: 4

Prep Time: 30 Min

CookTime: 10 Mim

Ingredients:

- ⅓ cup grated organic Parmesan cheese
- 4 cups shredded low-moisture organic mozzarella cheese
- 5 large free-range egg yolks
- 3 tablespoons Ghee
- 5 grape tomatoes
- 1 cup fresh basil leaves
- 2 tablespoons pine nuts
- 2 garlic cloves, peeled
- 1 Brazil nut
- Pinch ground nutmeg
- ¼ cup plus 2 teaspoons extra-virgin olive oil, divided

Instructions:

1. Using a mortar and pestle, coarsely grind the nut, nutmeg, basil, pine nuts, garlic, and Brazil with olive oil then mix in the Parmesan cheese. Set aside.
2. In a microwave-safe bowl, microwave the mozzarella until it is melted then add the egg yolks to the mozzarella and hand-knead.
3. Get a piece of parchment paper then roll out the dough. Refrigerate for 10 minutes.
4. In the meantime, boil salted water over high heat.
5. Using a knife, cut each roll into pieces. Together, drop the pieces into the boiling salted water.
6. Cook the gnocchi for 2 to 3 minutes then drain.
7. In a pan, melt the ghee on a medium-high heat. Add the gnocchi to the pan and fry for 1 minute.
8. In a separate pan, heat the remaining olive oil on a medium heat then add the tomatoes. Once softened, add in the pesto sauce just until warm.

9. Pour the tomatoes and pesto over the gnocchi
    and toss to combine. Heat for 1 more minute.
10. Serve and enjoy!

SNACKS

RECIPES

LOW-CARB NACHOS

Serving: 2 to 4

PrepTime: 10 min and 1hourtorest

CookTime: 15 min

Ingredients:

- 1½ teaspoons freshly squeezed lime juice
- Sea salt
- Freshly ground black pepper
- 1 bag pork rinds
- 2 cups shredded organic Cheddar cheese
- 1 medium tomato, seeded and chopped
- ¼ white onion, chopped
- 1 tablespoon chopped fresh cilantro
- 1 jalapeño pepper, seeded and minced
- 1 teaspoon minced garlic

Instructions:

1. In a bowl, mix together the tomato, cilantro, jalapeño onion, and garlic.

2. Add in the lime juice then season with salt and pepper.

3. Set the salsa aside for at least 1 hour.

4. After an hour, drain any excess liquid from the salsa.

5. Preheat the oven to 350°F.

6. Prepare a rimmed baking sheet with parchment paper or aluminum foil.

7. Spread out the pork rinds in a single layer on the sheet. Sprinkle the cheese on the pork rinds then top with salsa.

8. Bake the nachos for 15 minutes or until the cheese melts.

9. Serve hot and enjoy!

CREAMY DEVILED EGGS

Serving: 6

Prep Time: 10 Min

CookTime: 30 Min

Ingredients:

- 1 tablespoon dried dill
- 1 teaspoon sea salt
- 12 large free-range eggs
- 6 tablespoons mayonnaise

Instructions:

1. Place each whole egg in the cup of a muffin tin.
2. Turn the oven to 325°F and place the muffin tin in the oven.
3. Bake the eggs for 30 minutes.
4. Prepare a large bowl of ice water.
5. Transfer the eggs to the ice water and shake so they'll slightly crack each other.
6. Peel the eggsthen cut them in half. Get the yolks and put it in a small bowl.
7. Add the mayonnaise, dill, and salt to the bowl with the yolks then mix together until smooth.

8. Place the egg yolk mixture in a small zip lock plastic bag.

9. Cut off the corner of the bag at the bottom and pipe the filling into the egg halves.

10. Serve and enjoy!

CRAB DIP

Serving: 4 to 6

Prep Time: 10 Min

CookTime: 30 Min

Ingredients:

- 1 tablespoon mayonnaise
- 1 tablespoon horseradish
- 2 teaspoons Cajun seasoning
- ⅛ teaspoon garlic salt
- Grass-fed butter, at room temperature
- 1 pound lump crabmeat
- ½ cup diced red bell pepper
- 1 cup organic cream cheese, at room temperature

Instructions:

1. Preheat the oven to 350°F.
2. Grease a baking dish with butter.
3. In a bowl, mix the mayonnaise, horseradish, crabmeat, cream cheese, Cajun seasoning,

red bell pepper, and garlic salt until well
blended.

4. Transfer the dip to the baking dish and bake for
30 minutes.

5. Serve warm and enjoy!

BAKED PARMESAN CHIPS

Serving: 4

Prep Time: 5 Min

CookTime: 5 Min

Ingredients:

- 10 ounces shredded organic Parmesan cheese
- Sea salt

Instructions

1. Preheat the oven to 350°F.
2. Prepare a rimmed baking sheet with parchment paper.
3. Form a small Parmesan cheese circles on the sheet.
4. Bake for 3 to 5 minutes or until the cheese browns.
5. Once cooked, sprinkle the cheese with the salt.
6. Let cool before serving.

LOW-CARB MOZZARELLA CRUST PIZZA

Serving: 2
Prep Time: 5 Min
CookTime: 15 Min

Ingredients:

- ½ cup tomato sauce
- Grated organic Parmesan cheese
- 2 cups shredded organic mozzarella cheese
- 1 teaspoon garlic powder
- 1 teaspoon plus a pinch pizza seasoning, divided

Instructions:

1. Preheat the oven to 400°F.
2. Prepare a rimmed baking sheet with parchment paper.
3. Arrange the mozzarella on the baking sheet in an even layer to form a large rectangle.

4. Sprinkle the pinch of pizza seasoning and garlic powder on the cheese.
5. Bake for 12 to 15 minutes or until the cheese is melted.
6. Remove the baking sheet from the oven and let it cool for 3 minutes.
7. Spread the tomato sauce on the crust then sprinkle it with the Parmesan cheese and the remaining pizza seasoning.
8. Put the pizza back to the oven for 1 minute then slice and serve hot.

BAKED SOUR CREAM AND ONION PORK RINDS

Serving: 4 to 6

Prep Time: 20 Min

CookTime: 2½ Hours

Ingredients:

- 2 tablespoons onion powder
- 1 tablespoon garlic powder
- 2 pounds pork skin
- 3 tablespoons dried chives
- 3 tablespoons sweet cream buttermilk powder

Instructions:

1. Preheat the oven to 350°F.
2. Prepare a rimmed baking sheet with parchment paper.
3. Use a kitchen shearsto cut the pork skin into squares then place them all on the baking sheet.
4. Bake the skins for 2 to 3 hours.

5. Remove the baking sheet from the oven. Let it
    cool for few minutes.

6. In a bowl, mix the warm pork rinds with the
    chives, garlic powder, onion powder, and
    buttermilk powder.

7. Serve warm and enjoy!

MOZZARELLA STICKS

Serving: 4

PrepTime: 10 min and 1 hourtofreeze

CookTime: 2 min

Ingredients:

- 1 large free-range egg
- 1 large free-range egg white
- 10 whole-milk organic mozzarella cheese sticks
- Oil, for frying
- 1 bag pork rinds
- 1 tablespoon Italian seasoning
- 1 teaspoon garlic powder
- ¼ teaspoon sea salt
- ¼ teaspoon freshly ground black pepper
- ¼ cup grated organic Parmesan cheese

Instructions:

1. Prepare a rimmed baking sheet or a plate with parchment paper.

2. In a blender, combine the pork rinds, salt, and pepper, Italian seasoning, and garlic powder.
3. Transfer the mixture to a bowl.
4. In another bowl, whisk together the egg and egg white.
5. Cut each mozzarella stick into two.
6. Dip each mozzarella into the egg mixture and roll it in the breading.
7. Place the coated mozzarella sticks on the baking sheet or plate with parchment paper.
8. Freeze the mozzarella sticks for 45mins to 1 hour.
9. Get a pan and put it on a medium heat then fry the sticks for 1 minute on each side.
10. Serve warmand enjoy!

MINI SALAMI CHEESE PIZZAS

Serving: 1

Prep Time: 5 Min

CookTime: 1 Min

Ingredients:

- Pizza seasoning
- 4 slices Genoa salami
- 4 tablespoons Marinara Sauce, divided
- 4 tablespoons shredded organic mozzarella cheese, divided

Instructions:

1. Preheat the oven to broil.
2. Prepare a rimmed baking sheet with parchment paper.
3. Lay out the salami slices on the baking sheet.
4. Top each with a spoon of marinara sauce then sprinkle your preferred amount of mozzarella on each pizza and add a pinch of pizza seasoning.

5. Place the pizzas under the broiler forat least 1 minute.

6. Serve and enjoy!

BACON WHISKEY CARAMELIZED ONION DIP

Serving: 4 to 6

PrepTime: 10 min and 2 hoursto chill

CookTime: 25 Min

Ingredients:

- 1 cup organic sour cream
- ½ cup organic cream cheese, at room temperature
- ½ teaspoon sea salt
- 2 tablespoons bacon fat
- 3 teaspoons whiskey, divided
- 3 tablespoons water, divided
- ¼ teaspoon garlic powder
- 2 onions, halved lengthwise and cut crosswise into ¼-inch-thick slices

Instructions:

1. In a pan, melt the bacon fat over medium heat then add the onions and cook for 3 minutes.

2. When the onions begin to stick on the pan, stir in 1 teaspoon of whiskey then add 1 tablespoon of water. Repeat this until you've used all the whiskey.
3. Once the onions are soft and brown, transfer them to a bowl and refrigerate until cold.
4. In a blender, combine the garlic powder, sour cream, cream cheese, and salt. Blend them together until smooth.
5. Get the cold onions and to the blender. Transfer the dip to a container and refrigerate for 45minutes to 1 hour.
6. Stir the dip before serving.
7. Serve and enjoy!

ROASTED PESTO POPPERS

Serving: 6
Prep Time: 10 Min
CookTime: 20 Min

Ingredients:

- ¼ cup organic cream cheese, at room temperature
- 2 tablespoons diced shallot
- 1 teaspoon cayenne pepper sauce
- 1 tablespoon fresh thyme leaves
- 12 mini bell peppers, halved lengthwise and seeded
- ½ cup prepared pesto
- ¼ cup organic goat cheese

Instructions:

1. Preheat the oven to 350°F.
2. Prepare a rimmed baking sheet with parchment paper.
3. Lay the mini pepper halveson the sheet.

4. In a bowl, mix the pesto, shallot, cayenne
    pepper sauce, goat cheese, and cream
    cheese.
5. Fill the pepper with the pesto and cheese
    mixture.
6. Sprinkle them with thyme.
7. Bake for 20 to 25 minutes.
8. Serve hot and enjoy!

DESSERTS
RECIPES

BLACK FOREST PUDDING

Serving: 4

Prep Time: 10 Min

CookTime: 20 Min

Ingredients:

- Pinch sea salt
- 2 large free-range egg yolks
- 1 cup organic heavy cream
- 1 cup unsweetened almond milk
- 3 cherries, pitted and chopped
- ½ cup unsweetened cocoa powder
- ¼ cup Sugar-Free Vanilla Bean Sweetener

Instructions:

1. In a saucepan, heat the heavy cream, cherries, cocoa powderalmond milk, and salt over medium heat for 3 minutes. Remove the cherries and set aside.
2. In a bowl, beat the egg yolks. While whisking, pour the hot cream mixture into the eggs.
3. Pour the mixture back and cook. Stir consistentlyto scrape the sides and bottom of

the pot for 10 to 15 minutes. Once it thickened, put in the sweetener.

4. Transfer the mixture to a container and refrigerate for 2 hours.

5. Get the mixture then transfer to an ice-cream makerand just follow the manufacturer's instructions.

6. Once the ice cream is ready, fold in the cherries then put in acontainer and freeze for3 hours.

BERRY-SAGE FRUIT SALAD

Serving: 1

PrepTime: 5 Min

Ingredients:

- 1 large fresh sage leaf, chopped
- 1 teaspoon freshly squeezed Meyer lemon juice
- 1 teaspoon Sugar-Free Vanilla Bean Sweetener
- ½ cup blackberries
- ½ cup raspberries
- ¼ cup sliced strawberries
- 1 tablespoon blueberries

Instructions:

1. In a bowl, mix together all the ingredients and serve.

RICOTTA AND ALMOND DOUGHNUTS

Serving: 6

Prep Time: 10 Min

CookTime: 12 Min

Ingredients:

- Ghee
- ½ teaspoon ground cinnamon
- 2 ounces unsweetened chocolate
- 2 tablespoons unsalted grass-fed butter
- 2 tablespoons Sugar-Free Vanilla Bean Sweetener
- Your preferred sweetener to taste
- ¼ cup organic ricotta cheese
- 2 large free-range eggs
- 2 tablespoons almond flour
- 1 tablespoon coconut flour
- 1 teaspoon baking powder

Instructions:

1. Preheat the oven to 350°F.
2. Put ghee on a mini-doughnut pan.
3. In a blender, blend the ricotta cheese, eggs, cinnamon, almond flour, baking powder, and coconut flour until smooth.
4. Pour the butter into the doughnut cups.
5. Bake for 10 to 12 minutes or until the toothpick inserted in the centercomes out clean.
6. Remove the doughnuts from the tin and let them cool for a while.
7. In a microwave-safe bowl, combine the butter, chocolate, and sweeteners.
8. Microwave on high with a 20-second intervals. Stir well to melt the chocolate and thoroughly mix the ingredients.
9. Frost the cooled mini doughnuts.

LOW-CARB STRAWBERRIES AND CREAM CAKE

Serving: 1
Prep Time: 10 Min
CookTime: 4 Min

Ingredients:

- ¼ cup almond flour
- 4 strawberries, hulled and cut into chunks
- ¼ cup Whipped Cream
- 2 large free-range eggs
- ¼ cup Sugar-Free Vanilla Bean Sweetener
- 2 tablespoons Ghee, melted
- 2 tablespoons organic cream cheese

Instructions:

1. In a blender, blend the ghee, eggs, sweetener, and cream cheese.
2. Pourthe mixture into a small bowl.
3. Add in the almond flour and strawberries.

4. Microwave the butter on high for 4 to 5
    minutes.

5. Let the cake cool for 1 minute then top it with
    the whipped cream.

LEMON CURD TARTS

Serving: 6

Prep Time: 20 Min

CookTime: 20 Min

OvernighttoChill

Ingredients:

- ¾ cup almond meal
- ½ cup freshly squeezed lemon juice
- ¼ cup Sugar-Free Vanilla Bean Sweetener
- 4 large free-range egg yolks
- Grated zest of 3 lemons
- ½ cup plus 3 tablespoons unsalted grass-fed butter, melted, divided

Instructions:

1. Prepare a mini-muffin tin with parchment cups.
2. In a bowl, stir 3 tablespoons of melted butter into the almond meal.
3. Press the crust to the bottoms of the muffin cups.

4. In a blender, blend the egg yolks, sweetener, lemon zest and juice, and the remaining melted butter until smooth.

5. Transfer the filling to a saucepan thencook over low heat while stirring constantly for 15 minutes.

6. Pour the filling into the muffin cups then cover with plastic wrap and refrigerate overnight.

STRAWBERRIES MASCARPONE CREAM CHEESE

Serving: 3

PrepTime: 15 min and 30 mintochill

Ingredients:

- ¼ cup organic cream cheese
- 2 tablespoons organic mascarpone
- ¼ cup almond meal
- 10 small or 5 large strawberries
- 1 tablespoon Sugar-Free Vanilla Bean Sweetener

Instructions:

1. Put the almond meal on a plate or in a bowl.
2. Using a small melon baller, scoop out some of the strawberry's flesh from inside to fill.
3. In a microwave-safe bowl, microwave the mascarpone and cream cheese untilit melts. Stir to mix thoroughly then add in the sweetener.

4. Transfer the filling to a zip lock plastic bag and cut off a small piece of the corner at the bottom.

5. Pipe the filling into the strawberries then gently press the top of each strawberry into the almond flour.

6. Place the strawberries in a container and refrigerate for 25 to 30 minutes before serving.

PUMPKIN CHEESECAKE MUG PIE

Serving: 1

Prep Time: 10 min and 3 hourstochill

Ingredients:

- 1 tablespoon Sugar-Free Vanilla Bean Sweetener
- ⅛ teaspoon pumpkin pie spice
- Pinch nutmeg
- 2 tablespoons almond meal
- 4½ teaspoons unsalted grass-fed butter, divided
- ¼ cup organic cream cheese, at room temperature
- 2 tablespoons organic heavy cream
- 2 tablespoons pure pumpkin purée

Instructions:

1. In a microwave-safe mug, combine the almond meal and the butter then microwave on high for 30 seconds.

2. Mix the butter and almond meal together then flatten the mixture into the bottom of the mug to form a crust.

3. In a bowl, mix together the cream cheese, heavy cream, pumpkin, pumpkin pie spice, sweetener, and the remaining butter.

4. Transfer the mixture into the mug then sprinkle it with a little nutmeg and refrigerate for 3 hours.

MINI COCONUT PIES

Serving: 12

PrepTime: 10 min and 30 min to chill

CookTime: 10 min

Ingredients:

- 3 tablespoons Sugar-Free Vanilla Bean Sweetener
- 1 cup unsweetened coconut cream
- ¼ cup unsweetened shredded coconut
- 1 tablespoon coconut oil
- 1 cup coconut flour
- 2 large free-range eggs
- ½ cup Ghee, melted

Instructions:

1. Preheat the oven to 350°F.
2. Putthe coconut oil in the cups of mini-muffin tin.
3. In a bowl, whisk together the coconut flour, eggs, ghee, and sweetener.
4. Divide the flour mixture between the muffin cups then pat into the bottom of each cup.

5. Bake for 10 minutes.

6. Let it cool then remove the little coconut pie
    shells from the tin.

7. In a bowl, combine the shredded coconut,
    coconut cream, and the remaining sweetener
    and then mix thoroughly.

8. Top each pie with cream mixture then chill for
    at least 30 minutes before serving.

PEANUT BUTTER AND AVOCADO BOMBS

Serving: 6

PrepTime: 10 min and 3 hoursto freeze

Ingredients:

- 1 cup peanut butter, smooth or chunky
- 1 avocado, peeled, pitted, and chopped
- 1 tablespoon Sugar-Free Vanilla Bean Sweetener
- ½ cup coconut oil, melted
- ½ cup Ghee, melted
- 3 tablespoons organic heavy cream

Instructions:

1. Prepare a 12-cup tin with parchment paper.
2. In a blender, combine the coconut oil, ghee, heavy cream, avocado, peanut butter and sweetener. Blend all ingredients until smooth.
3. Pour the mixture into the parchment papers and freeze for 3 hours before serving.

About The Author

The Health Buff is a group of writers that aims to help people on what diet they want to achieve. They explore a lot of dishes from different parts of the world and share them by putting everything into a book. These writers specifically share the diets and food that just actually worked for them.

The Health Buff writers are all food and health enthusiasts, thus, coming up with the idea of sharing what they all love to do to inspire other people look after their health. They all believed that the best investment that you can ever make is in your own HEALTH.